AI Chronic Disease Prevention

How AI Identifies Hidden Health Risks Early to Reduce Long-Term Disease Burden

By Joe Correa

Published by Live Stronger Faster

This book is for educational and informational purposes only. The author and publisher are not engaged in rendering legal, financial, or other professional advice. Readers should consult a qualified professional before making any financial decisions.

First Edition

Table of Contents

Introduction

Aging does not suddenly begin at forty, fifty, or sixty, and chronic disease does not arrive overnight. It develops quietly, often years or decades before symptoms appear, shaped by small biological changes that accumulate beneath the surface. For most people, the first sign of chronic illness is not an early warning but a diagnosis—hypertension discovered during a routine visit, blood sugar levels that have crossed into diabetes, joint pain that no longer fades, or fatigue that refuses to lift. By the time these conditions are identified, the body has already adapted to dysfunction, making reversal far more difficult. This book exists because that traditional timeline is no longer inevitable. Artificial intelligence now makes it possible to detect risk long before disease takes hold, transforming aging from a reactive experience into a proactive, informed, and controllable process.

Chronic diseases account for the majority of health decline after midlife, yet most are not caused by sudden failure. They emerge from patterns—subtle shifts in inflammation, metabolic efficiency, hormonal signaling, cardiovascular strain, immune resilience, and cellular repair. Historically, medicine has struggled to track these patterns in real time because the data is complex, scattered, and highly individualized. Human clinicians excel at diagnosis once thresholds are crossed, but they are not designed to continuously analyze thousands of micro-signals across months and years. Artificial intelligence changes this limitation fundamentally. AI systems can process massive volumes of health data simultaneously, detect deviations long before they meet diagnostic criteria, and reveal personal risk trajectories that would otherwise remain invisible. This book explains how that shift works and how it can be used responsibly to reduce long-term disease burden as you age.

For adults over forty, chronic disease prevention becomes the most important health strategy, even if you feel well today. This stage of life is often when biological resilience begins to decline quietly while external responsibilities increase. Careers, family obligations, financial pressure, and time constraints often push health into the background. Unfortunately, this is also the period when early markers of cardiovascular disease, insulin resistance, neurodegeneration, autoimmune imbalance, and musculoskeletal decline begin to emerge. Traditional healthcare models focus on treating conditions after they are measurable and billable, not when they are preventable. AI-driven health analysis introduces a different framework—one that prioritizes early pattern recognition, individualized risk assessment, and intervention timing that aligns with your unique biology rather than population averages. This book does not position artificial intelligence as a replacement for doctors, medications, or common-sense lifestyle practices. Instead, it presents AI as an intelligence layer that sits above traditional healthcare, integrating data from lab work, wearable devices, medical history, genetics, lifestyle inputs, and longitudinal trends to provide clarity that was previously unattainable. AI excels at connecting dots across systems—linking sleep quality to inflammation, glucose variability to cognitive fatigue, gait stability to neurological risk, or heart rate variability to immune stress. These connections matter because chronic disease rarely affects only one system at a time. It is systemic by nature, and prevention requires systemic awareness.

One of the most powerful advantages of AI in chronic disease prevention is its ability to personalize risk. Two individuals of the same age with similar lab results can have vastly different long-term outcomes depending on how their bodies respond to stress, recover from exertion, process nutrients, and regulate inflammation. AI models trained on diverse datasets can identify which markers matter most for you specifically, rather than relying on generalized thresholds that may not reflect your real risk. This shifts prevention from a generic checklist to a living, adaptive strategy that evolves as your body changes. In this book, you will learn how AI interprets these patterns and how to use that insight without becoming overwhelmed or dependent on technology. Chronic disease prevention is often misunderstood as an all-or-nothing pursuit, requiring extreme diets, aggressive supplementation, or constant monitoring. In reality, the most effective prevention strategies are incremental and sustainable, guided by feedback rather than fear. AI supports this approach by identifying which changes produce meaningful improvements and which are unnecessary. Instead of guessing whether a new habit is helping, AI can show measurable impact over time, reinforcing consistency and reducing burnout. This is especially important after forty, when recovery slows and excess intervention can backfire. Prevention must respect the body's limits while strengthening its adaptive capacity, and AI provides the feedback loop that makes this balance possible.

As you move through your fifties and beyond, the goal of chronic disease prevention expands. It is no longer just about avoiding diagnosis but about preserving quality of life, independence, and confidence in your body's reliability. Conditions such as cardiovascular disease, type 2 diabetes, arthritis, osteoporosis, neurodegenerative disorders, and chronic fatigue syndromes often intersect, compounding their effects. AI systems can model these interactions, identifying upstream drivers that influence multiple conditions simultaneously. Addressing these root factors early—such as chronic inflammation, mitochondrial dysfunction, sleep disruption, or autonomic imbalance—can reduce risk across several disease pathways at once. This book will guide you through that systems-level perspective in a way that is practical and actionable.

Another critical theme of this book is timing. Intervention too late requires aggressive treatment, while intervention too early without clear signals can create unnecessary anxiety. AI helps identify the optimal window—the point at which small adjustments yield the greatest long-term benefit. This is where chronic disease prevention becomes efficient rather than exhausting. By learning how AI identifies inflection points in health data, you gain the ability to act with precision instead of urgency. The result is a calmer, more confident relationship with your health, grounded in evidence rather than guesswork.

Ethics and responsibility are also central to any discussion of AI and health. Data privacy, algorithmic bias, over-reliance on automated recommendations, and misinformation are legitimate concerns. This book addresses these issues directly, emphasizing informed use rather than blind trust. You will learn how to interpret AI-generated insights, ask better questions of your healthcare providers, and maintain agency over your decisions. The purpose of AI is not to dictate your choices but to illuminate options that align with your goals and values. When used correctly, it enhances human judgment rather than replacing it. This volume fits into the larger **AI Longevity for 40+, 50+, 60+** series by focusing on prevention as the foundation of all other longevity strategies. Muscle preservation, bone health, heart optimization, mobility, and energy restoration all depend on minimizing chronic disease burden. Without early detection and intervention, efforts in these areas become reactive and limited. By understanding how AI identifies hidden risks early, you strengthen every other aspect of aging well. This book prepares you to engage with the rest of the series from a position of foresight rather than damage control.

Ultimately, **AI Chronic Disease Prevention** is about reclaiming time—time free from unnecessary illness, time spent active rather than managing symptoms, and time invested in life rather than recovery. Aging will always involve change, but decline is not inevitable. With the intelligence now available, you can see further down the road than any generation before you. This book is your guide to using that visibility wisely, building a future where health is monitored quietly in the background while life remains fully in the foreground.

Chapter 1

Why Chronic Disease Rarely Starts Where It's Diagnosed

Chronic disease is almost never a sudden event. It does not begin on the day a doctor delivers a diagnosis, nor does it appear the moment symptoms become uncomfortable enough to demand attention. Instead, chronic disease unfolds slowly, quietly, and predictably through a series of biological compromises that accumulate over time. These compromises often go unnoticed because they remain below the threshold of pain, dysfunction, or abnormal lab values. By the time disease is officially identified, the body has already adapted to long-term imbalance, making treatment more complex and recovery more limited. Understanding this hidden timeline is the first step toward prevention, and it is where artificial intelligence fundamentally changes what is possible for aging adults.

The human body is designed to compensate. When blood sugar regulation weakens, the body adjusts insulin signaling. When inflammation rises, tissues adapt by altering immune responses. When cardiovascular efficiency declines, circulation reroutes and pressure increases. These adaptations allow daily life to continue, masking the early stages of disease.

Traditional healthcare systems are built to identify failure once compensation breaks down, not while it is still quietly functioning. This is why so many adults are shocked by diagnoses that seem to appear "out of nowhere." In reality, the warning signs were present for years, but they were dispersed across systems and time in ways that exceeded human analytical capacity.

Most chronic diseases share common upstream drivers. Low-grade inflammation, mitochondrial inefficiency, hormonal dysregulation, impaired glucose metabolism, sleep disruption, and nervous system imbalance all interact to create conditions where disease can thrive. These drivers do not progress linearly. They fluctuate based on stress, nutrition, activity, environment, and recovery. Because of this variability, short-term snapshots such as annual blood tests often miss the pattern. Artificial intelligence excels precisely where human observation struggles: it identifies trends across time, correlations across systems, and deviations from personal baselines rather than population averages.

One of the most damaging myths about chronic disease is that it is primarily genetic or inevitable with age. Genetics influence risk, but they rarely dictate outcomes on their own. What matters far more is how genes interact with lifestyle, environment, and biological stressors over decades. AI models trained on large-scale longitudinal data can identify how these interactions unfold in real life, revealing that many so-called "age-related" diseases are actually acceleration-related diseases. They progress faster when early signals are ignored and slow dramatically when those signals are addressed in time.

After the age of forty, the body's margin for error narrows. Recovery takes longer, inflammation resolves more slowly, and metabolic flexibility decreases. These changes do not mean decline is unavoidable, but they do mean that early misalignments carry greater consequences. AI-driven health systems recognize this shift and adjust expectations accordingly. Instead of asking whether a lab value is technically normal, AI evaluates whether it is optimal for your age, trajectory, and historical pattern. This distinction is critical. Many chronic diseases develop while values remain "normal," but trends are moving in the wrong direction.

Chronic disease also rarely exists in isolation. Cardiovascular risk influences cognitive health. Insulin resistance affects joint inflammation. Poor sleep accelerates immune dysfunction. Traditional medicine often treats these issues separately because they appear in different specialties, but AI views the body as a single, interconnected system. By modeling interactions across organs and processes, AI can identify leverage points where small interventions produce outsized benefits. This systems-level insight allows prevention strategies to be efficient rather than overwhelming, focusing effort where it matters most.

Another limitation of conventional disease prevention is timing. Advice is often delivered either too late, when damage has accumulated, or too early and generically, leading to confusion or disengagement. AI narrows this gap by identifying inflection points—moments when biological trends begin to diverge meaningfully from healthy trajectories. Acting at these points requires less effort and produces more durable results. This is not about constant monitoring or anxiety-driven optimization. It is about informed awareness and timely action guided by evidence rather than fear.

The role of AI in chronic disease prevention is not prediction in the dramatic sense, but probability management. It does not declare that disease will occur; it reveals how likely it is under current conditions and how that likelihood changes with intervention. This reframes health from a fixed destiny to a dynamic process that responds to informed choices. For adults in midlife and beyond, this shift restores a sense of agency that is often lost after diagnosis. Prevention becomes a partnership between technology, biology, and human judgment.

Importantly, AI does not replace clinical care. It enhances it by providing context that clinicians rarely have time or tools to assemble. When AI insights are used responsibly, they improve conversations with healthcare providers, sharpen decision-making, and reduce unnecessary interventions. This chapter establishes the foundation for understanding why chronic disease is detectable long before it is diagnosable and why AI is uniquely suited to reveal those early signals. In the chapters that follow, you will learn how specific systems—metabolic, cardiovascular, neurological, musculoskeletal, and immune—can be monitored and supported using this approach to reduce disease burden as you age.

The Years Before the Diagnosis

When Mark turned forty-eight, he considered himself healthy. He worked full-time, exercised a few times a week, and had no major medical issues. His annual physicals were unremarkable, his blood pressure was "a little high but nothing concerning," and his cholesterol was "borderline." He accepted these comments as normal for his age and moved on. Like many people, he believed chronic disease was something that happened later, to others, and mostly due to bad luck or genetics. His father had developed heart disease in his sixties, but Mark assumed modern medicine would catch anything serious in time.

What Mark did not notice was how his energy had slowly changed. He woke up feeling less refreshed, needed more caffeine to stay focused, and recovered more slowly from workouts. He attributed this to stress and aging. His sleep tracker showed inconsistent rest, but he rarely looked at the data beyond total hours. His diet fluctuated with work demands, and his activity level declined during busy months. None of these changes felt dramatic enough to warrant concern. They were small, manageable, and easy to ignore.

At fifty-one, Mark's company offered a voluntary wellness program that included access to an AI-driven health platform. Skeptical but curious, he enrolled. The system integrated his wearable data, historical lab results, lifestyle inputs, and family history. Within weeks, it identified patterns he had never been shown before. His heart rate variability had been declining steadily for years, indicating reduced autonomic resilience. His fasting glucose remained normal, but post-meal variability suggested early insulin resistance. Inflammatory markers fluctuated in response to poor sleep, and these fluctuations correlated with cognitive fatigue and joint stiffness he had dismissed as normal.

The platform did not alarm him or predict disease. Instead, it showed trajectories. If his patterns continued unchanged, his probability of developing cardiovascular disease and metabolic syndrome within the next decade was significantly higher than average for his age. More importantly, it showed which factors mattered most for him. Improving sleep consistency, reducing late-night stress, adjusting meal timing, and moderating training intensity produced measurable improvements within weeks. Mark did not overhaul his life. He made targeted changes informed by feedback rather than vague advice.

Over the next two years, Mark continued to monitor trends rather than chase perfection. His clinician reviewed the AI summaries during appointments and adjusted recommendations accordingly. His blood pressure stabilized without medication, inflammatory markers decreased, and energy returned gradually. When a colleague his age was diagnosed with type 2 diabetes, Mark realized how close he might have been to the same path. The difference was not discipline or luck, but visibility. He had seen the years before the diagnosis and acted while the body was still adaptable.

By the time Mark turned fifty-five, his health profile looked better than it had a decade earlier. He had not avoided aging, but he had avoided unnecessary decline. Chronic disease had not disappeared as a concept; it had been displaced from inevitability. The AI system did not save him in a dramatic moment. It simply revealed what had always been happening and gave him time to respond. That time, he would later say, was the most valuable gift he had received.

Chapter 2

The Silent Signals AI Detects Long Before Chronic Disease Appears

Chronic disease does not begin with pain, diagnosis, or dysfunction. It begins with subtle signals—small deviations in biological patterns that the human body compensates for quietly and efficiently. These signals rarely trigger alarms in traditional healthcare because they exist in relationships rather than absolutes. A blood marker may be technically "normal" while its trend over time is concerning. A symptom may appear occasionally, not frequently enough to report, yet consistently enough to matter. Artificial intelligence is uniquely capable of identifying these silent signals because it does not rely on single data points or subjective interpretation. It evaluates patterns, correlations, and trajectories across time, revealing early warnings that precede chronic disease by years.

One of the most important signals AI detects is loss of biological resilience. Resilience refers to how quickly and effectively the body returns to baseline after stress, whether that stress is physical exertion, poor sleep, emotional strain, illness, or dietary disruption. As people age, resilience naturally declines, but accelerated loss of resilience is a powerful predictor of future disease. AI systems analyze recovery curves rather than static measurements, identifying when the body begins to struggle with stress it once handled easily. This decline often appears long before traditional markers cross diagnostic thresholds, making it one of the earliest and most actionable signals of future risk.

Inflammation is another silent signal that AI detects with far greater precision than conventional methods. Chronic low-grade inflammation fluctuates daily and responds to lifestyle, environment, and internal stressors. Single lab tests often miss its significance because values rise and fall within acceptable ranges. AI identifies inflammatory volatility rather than isolated elevation, revealing patterns that suggest immune dysregulation rather than temporary response. This distinction matters because persistent inflammatory instability is a common upstream driver of cardiovascular disease, metabolic disorders, joint degeneration, neurodegeneration, and autoimmune conditions.

Metabolic flexibility is a third critical signal. This refers to the body's ability to efficiently switch between fuel sources and regulate blood sugar in response to food, activity, and rest. AI analyzes glucose variability, insulin response patterns, energy levels, and recovery timing to assess metabolic health beyond fasting values. Loss of metabolic flexibility often precedes diabetes and cardiovascular disease by many years, yet it is rarely identified early because symptoms are subtle and intermittent. AI recognizes when these patterns begin to drift, allowing intervention before damage accumulates.

Sleep architecture provides another powerful early warning. Poor sleep is often dismissed as a lifestyle inconvenience rather than a biological signal. AI systems analyze sleep stages, fragmentation, timing consistency, and recovery impact to determine whether sleep disruption is transient or systemic. Chronic sleep instability affects hormone regulation, immune function, cognitive health, and cardiovascular resilience. When AI detects persistent degradation in sleep quality correlated with other biological stress markers, it signals elevated chronic disease risk even if the individual reports feeling "fine."

Cardiovascular signals extend far beyond blood pressure and cholesterol. AI evaluates heart rate variability, resting heart rate trends, exertion response, and recovery efficiency to assess autonomic balance and vascular health. Small but consistent changes in these patterns often indicate early cardiovascular strain long before structural disease develops. These signals are particularly valuable because cardiovascular dysfunction frequently underlies or accelerates other chronic conditions. Detecting these changes early allows prevention strategies to protect multiple systems simultaneously. Neurological and cognitive signals are equally subtle. AI can correlate reaction time, focus consistency, sleep quality, mood variability, and stress response to identify early signs of cognitive overload or neuroinflammatory stress. These patterns do not indicate disease on their own, but when combined with metabolic and cardiovascular data, they can reveal emerging risk for cognitive decline. Traditional healthcare rarely integrates these domains, but AI thrives on such integration, recognizing risk profiles that are invisible when systems are viewed in isolation.

What makes these signals powerful is not their individual presence, but their interaction. Chronic disease emerges when multiple systems drift out of alignment together. AI detects convergence—when metabolic stress coincides with inflammatory instability, when sleep disruption aligns with autonomic imbalance, or when cognitive fatigue parallels vascular strain. These intersections represent tipping points where small adjustments can restore balance or neglect can accelerate decline. Recognizing these moments transforms prevention from guesswork into strategy.

Importantly, AI does not interpret these signals as destiny. It frames them as indicators of probability and direction. Trends can stabilize, improve, or worsen depending on response. This perspective shifts chronic disease prevention away from fear-based monitoring and toward informed stewardship.

Understanding the silent signals AI detects empowers individuals to act early without panic, preserving health quietly and efficiently. This chapter establishes the language and logic of early detection, preparing you to understand how AI translates invisible biological whispers into meaningful insight.

The Data She Almost Ignored

When Elena turned fifty-six, she felt healthy by every conventional measure. She worked part-time, walked daily, and rarely got sick. Her doctor visits were routine, and her lab results were consistently described as "within range." She slept reasonably well and maintained a balanced diet, though stress had become a constant presence since caring for her aging mother. Elena had never considered herself at risk for chronic disease. She assumed that serious health problems would announce themselves clearly, not quietly.

At her daughter's urging, Elena began using a health monitoring platform that integrated wearable data and historical records. She was initially unimpressed. The daily metrics felt abstract, and nothing seemed urgent. After several months, the system generated a summary highlighting patterns rather than warnings. It showed that her recovery from physical and emotional stress had slowed noticeably over the past three years. Her heart rate variability declined during periods of poor sleep and did not rebound as quickly as it once had. Glucose variability increased during stressful weeks, even though her fasting numbers remained normal.

Elena almost dismissed the report. She felt fine, after all. But curiosity led her to review the correlations. On weeks when her sleep was fragmented, her inflammation markers subtly increased. On days when she skipped walks due to caregiving demands, her metabolic stability dipped. None of these changes were dramatic, but together they formed a picture she had never seen before. Her body was compensating, but less efficiently each year.

With guidance from her clinician, Elena made small adjustments. She protected sleep timing more carefully, reduced evening stress exposure, and adjusted meal composition rather than calories. She did not chase perfection. She followed trends. Over the next year, the AI summaries showed gradual improvement. Recovery curves shortened. Inflammatory volatility decreased. Energy stabilized. When her mother passed away, the stress did not derail her health as it might have previously.

Two years later, Elena's close friend was diagnosed with rheumatoid arthritis after years of unexplained fatigue and joint stiffness. Elena recognized the path immediately. She realized how close she had been to dismissing the same early signals. Her health had not been preserved through vigilance or fear, but through attention. AI had not predicted disease; it had revealed direction. By listening early, Elena changed course without ever feeling like she was fighting illness. She was simply maintaining balance, one quiet adjustment at a time.

Chapter 3

How AI Turns Early Warnings Into Personalized Prevention Strategies

Early detection alone does not prevent chronic disease. Awareness without direction often leads to confusion, anxiety, or inaction. The true power of artificial intelligence in health lies in its ability to convert early biological signals into clear, prioritized, and personalized prevention strategies that align with how the body actually changes with age. This chapter explains how AI moves from observation to intervention, transforming invisible risk into practical action without overwhelming the individual or relying on extreme measures.

Traditional health advice is largely static. It offers general recommendations based on age brackets, averages, or population studies rather than individual biology. While these guidelines can be useful, they fail to account for how differently bodies respond to stress, recovery, nutrition, sleep, and aging. AI replaces static advice with adaptive guidance. It continuously evaluates incoming data, learns how a specific body reacts over time, and adjusts recommendations accordingly. This creates prevention strategies that evolve alongside the individual rather than becoming outdated or irrelevant. One of the most important functions AI performs is prioritization. The human body produces thousands of signals every day, and attempting to address all of them simultaneously is neither realistic nor effective. AI identifies which signals are upstream drivers rather than downstream consequences. For example, joint pain may appear to be a musculoskeletal issue, but AI may reveal that inflammatory instability driven by poor sleep and metabolic stress is the true source. Addressing sleep and glucose regulation in that case produces greater benefit than focusing solely on joints. This prioritization ensures effort is invested where it yields the greatest return.

AI also translates biological data into behavioral relevance. Instead of presenting abstract metrics, it reveals cause-and-effect relationships between daily choices and physiological outcomes. When an individual sees that irregular sleep timing directly precedes spikes in inflammation or reduced cognitive clarity, motivation becomes grounded in evidence rather than willpower. This feedback loop strengthens consistency without relying on fear or discipline. Prevention becomes intuitive because the body's responses are visible and understandable.

Another critical advantage of AI-driven prevention is precision timing. Intervening too aggressively when the body is stable can create unnecessary stress, while intervening too late requires more intensive correction. AI monitors trend velocity to determine when a pattern is stabilizing, drifting, or accelerating toward risk. This allows interventions to be scaled appropriately. Small course corrections applied early often prevent the need for medication or invasive treatment later, preserving autonomy and quality of life as people age.

AI also personalizes thresholds rather than relying on standardized cutoffs. Many chronic diseases develop while lab values remain technically normal. AI identifies deviation from an individual's historical baseline rather than population norms. This is especially important after midlife, when subtle declines accumulate gradually. By recognizing when a value is abnormal for a specific person rather than abnormal in general, AI enables earlier and more relevant action.

Importantly, AI does not prescribe rigid routines. It identifies ranges and patterns that support stability while allowing flexibility. Prevention strategies that demand perfection are rarely sustainable. AI-driven guidance respects variability, recognizing that occasional disruption is part of life. What matters is recovery efficiency and trend direction over time. This perspective reduces guilt and burnout while reinforcing behaviors that genuinely support long-term health.

AI also strengthens collaboration with healthcare providers. Rather than replacing clinical judgment, it supplies context that clinicians rarely have time to assemble. Longitudinal summaries, trend visualizations, and correlation insights improve decision-making and communication. This shared understanding shifts care from reactive treatment to proactive management, especially for individuals at elevated risk of chronic disease.

Ultimately, AI transforms prevention from guesswork into stewardship. It does not promise immunity from aging or illness, but it dramatically improves the odds of aging with fewer burdens and greater independence. By translating early signals into targeted, timely action, AI allows chronic disease prevention to occur quietly, efficiently, and sustainably. This chapter establishes how insight becomes strategy, setting the stage for applying AI across specific systems such as metabolism, cardiovascular health, mobility, cognition, and energy in the chapters ahead.

The Adjustments That Changed Everything

When Thomas turned sixty-two, he felt caught between two versions of himself. One part of him still believed he was healthy. He stayed active, maintained a reasonable weight, and rarely visited the doctor outside of routine appointments. The other part sensed subtle changes he could not explain. His energy dipped unpredictably, his joints felt stiffer after long days, and recovery from physical activity took longer than it once had. None of it seemed serious enough to worry about, but together it created an unease he struggled to name.

At his wife's encouragement, Thomas enrolled in a preventive health program that used AI to analyze long-term trends rather than isolated results. He expected to be told that everything was normal. Instead, the system showed patterns that surprised him. His inflammatory markers fluctuated more widely than they had a decade earlier, particularly after nights of poor sleep. His cardiovascular recovery after exertion slowed gradually year after year. His glucose levels remained normal, but variability increased during periods of stress. No single issue stood out, but the convergence of patterns suggested rising chronic disease risk.

What surprised Thomas most was the simplicity of the recommendations. The AI system did not ask him to overhaul his lifestyle. It identified two primary drivers of his instability: inconsistent sleep timing and overexertion without adequate recovery. Small adjustments were suggested. He shifted his workouts to earlier in the day, protected a consistent bedtime, and incorporated lighter recovery days instead of pushing through fatigue. He was skeptical that such modest changes could matter. Within months, the feedback was undeniable.

His recovery curves improved. Inflammatory volatility decreased. Energy stabilized. The stiffness he had accepted as age-related became less frequent. His clinician reviewed the AI summaries and agreed that medication was unnecessary at that stage. Prevention had worked not through intensity, but through precision.

Two years later, Thomas watched several friends navigate new diagnoses—hypertension, arthritis, metabolic disease. He recognized the path he might have followed had he ignored those early signals. His health had not been preserved by dramatic intervention, but by alignment. AI had not frightened him into action. It had shown him where to act and when to stop. Aging continued, but decline slowed quietly in the background, allowing life to remain in the foreground where it belonged.

Chapter 4

Why Early Intervention Works Better Than Late Treatment

The difference between prevention and treatment is not simply timing; it is biological leverage. When chronic disease is addressed early, the body is still adaptable, responsive, and capable of restoring balance with minimal force. When disease is addressed late, systems have already reorganized around dysfunction, making reversal slower, more complex, and often incomplete. Artificial intelligence enables early intervention not by accelerating treatment, but by identifying when the body still has the capacity to self-correct. This chapter explains why acting early produces disproportionate benefits and how AI identifies the narrow windows where small actions prevent large consequences.

The human body is built around compensation. When one system begins to falter, others adjust to maintain function. Blood vessels stiffen to preserve circulation, insulin secretion increases to manage rising glucose, inflammation escalates to repair recurring stress, and neural pathways reroute to preserve cognition. These compensations are effective in the short term, but costly over time. Chronic disease emerges when compensatory mechanisms become permanent. AI identifies the moment when compensation shifts from adaptive to destructive, long before symptoms force attention.

Late-stage treatment often targets downstream effects rather than upstream causes. Medications lower numbers, reduce pain, or suppress symptoms, but they rarely restore the underlying regulatory balance that was lost years earlier. Early intervention, by contrast, focuses on restoring regulation itself. AI reveals which regulatory systems are slipping and which behaviors or stressors are driving that shift. Addressing these factors early reduces the need for aggressive intervention later and preserves functional capacity across multiple systems.

One of the most misunderstood aspects of early intervention is that it does not require dramatic lifestyle change. In fact, extreme changes applied too early can increase stress and undermine resilience. AI-guided intervention emphasizes precision rather than intensity. It identifies minimal effective changes that produce measurable improvement, allowing the body to respond without being overwhelmed. This approach aligns with how aging bodies adapt best: gradually, consistently, and within tolerable limits.

AI also recognizes that intervention capacity changes with age. After forty, recovery slows. After fifty, redundancy decreases. After sixty, resilience depends heavily on stability. Early intervention respects these realities by acting before these constraints tighten further. Preventing disease at fifty is easier than reversing it at sixty-five. Preventing disease at forty-five is easier still. AI shifts the health conversation from urgency to foresight, encouraging action when the cost is lowest and the return is highest.

Another reason early intervention is so effective is that it prevents cascade failure. Chronic disease rarely affects one system alone. Metabolic dysfunction strains the cardiovascular system, which impacts cognitive health, which accelerates mobility decline. AI identifies these cascade pathways early, allowing intervention at the top rather than the bottom. Stopping a cascade before it begins preserves multiple systems simultaneously, reducing overall disease burden and complexity.

Psychologically, early intervention also changes the relationship people have with their health. Late treatment often arrives with fear, urgency, and loss of control. Early intervention arrives with clarity and agency. AI-driven insights are not alarms; they are maps. They show where the body is heading and how direction can be altered. This reduces anxiety and increases engagement because action feels purposeful rather than reactive. Importantly, early intervention does not eliminate the need for medical care. It enhances it. AI provides context that helps clinicians recommend proportionate responses rather than default escalation. When trends improve, intervention can ease. When trends worsen, escalation is justified. This dynamic approach reduces overtreatment while preventing neglect, aligning care with reality rather than rigid protocols.

Ultimately, early intervention works because it aligns with biology. Aging is not a cliff; it is a slope. AI allows that slope to be monitored, adjusted, and stabilized before it becomes steep. Chronic disease prevention is most effective when it is quiet, gradual, and almost unnoticeable. This chapter establishes why acting early is not about doing more, but about doing less at the right time, preserving health without turning life into a constant project.

The Window She Didn't Miss

When Karen turned fifty-nine, she felt caught between reassurance and concern. Her doctor told her her labs were acceptable, but added that "things tend to change quickly at this age." The comment stayed with her. She felt mostly well, yet recovery from long days felt slower, sleep less reliable, and aches more persistent. She feared becoming someone who waited until something broke before paying attention. Karen enrolled in a preventive health program that used AI to analyze trends across several years. The system did not identify disease. Instead, it highlighted a narrowing margin of resilience. Sleep disruption triggered inflammation more readily than before. Physical exertion produced longer recovery curves. Glucose variability increased during stressful weeks. None of it demanded treatment, but together it suggested that her body was nearing a tipping point.

What surprised Karen was how small the recommended adjustments were. She reduced late-night screen exposure, adjusted workout intensity, and spaced meals more consistently. These were changes she could sustain without resentment. Over time, the AI summaries showed stabilization. Recovery improved. Sleep became more predictable. Inflammation fluctuated less dramatically.

A year later, Karen's sister was diagnosed with hypertension and arthritis within months of each other. Watching the struggle, Karen realized how close she might have been to the same path. The difference was not genetics or discipline. It was timing. She had acted while her body could still respond easily.

At sixty-three, Karen remained active and independent. Aging had not stopped, but decline had slowed. She did not feel like she was managing illness. She felt like she was maintaining balance. The window she had acted within was narrow and quiet, but it made all the difference. AI had not saved her from disease in a dramatic moment. It had simply shown her when to move—and when moving was still easy.

Chapter 5

How AI Prevents Disease by Protecting the Body's Core Regulatory Systems

Chronic disease rarely begins with failure. It begins with loss of regulation. Long before organs deteriorate or symptoms emerge, the systems responsible for balance, adaptation, and recovery start to drift. These regulatory systems control how the body responds to stress, repairs damage, distributes energy, manages inflammation, and maintains internal stability. When they function well, aging remains gradual and manageable. When they weaken, disease accelerates quietly. Artificial intelligence excels at monitoring and protecting these regulatory systems, making it one of the most powerful tools ever developed for long-term disease prevention.

The most critical regulatory system is the autonomic nervous system, which governs heart rate, blood pressure, digestion, immune response, and stress adaptation. This system operates largely outside conscious control, adjusting constantly to internal and external demands. Chronic stress, poor sleep, metabolic strain, and aging itself gradually impair this system's flexibility. AI detects this impairment through changes in heart rate variability, recovery patterns, sleep architecture, and stress responsiveness. Protecting autonomic balance early prevents downstream consequences across nearly every chronic disease category.

Metabolic regulation is another core system where AI-driven prevention is transformative. Rather than focusing solely on glucose levels or weight, AI evaluates how efficiently the body processes fuel under varying conditions. Loss of metabolic flexibility strains blood vessels, accelerates inflammation, disrupts hormone signaling, and impairs cognitive function. AI identifies early metabolic inefficiencies before they harden into diabetes or cardiovascular disease, allowing intervention that restores balance instead of managing damage.

Inflammatory regulation plays a similarly central role. Inflammation is not inherently harmful; it is essential for repair and defense. Problems arise when inflammation becomes unstable, exaggerated, or persistent. AI distinguishes healthy inflammatory responses from chronic volatility by analyzing fluctuations rather than single measurements. This allows identification of immune stress long before autoimmune disease, arthritis, or neurodegeneration develops. Stabilizing inflammation early reduces risk across multiple systems simultaneously.

Sleep regulation is often underestimated despite its foundational role in health. Sleep is when regulatory systems reset, consolidate learning, repair tissues, and recalibrate hormones. AI monitors not just sleep duration, but timing consistency, fragmentation, stage distribution, and recovery impact. Chronic disruption to sleep regulation accelerates nearly every form of chronic disease. AI-driven insight allows sleep to be corrected as a regulatory priority rather than treated as a secondary lifestyle issue.

Hormonal regulation also shifts subtly with age. Changes in cortisol rhythm, insulin sensitivity, sex hormones, and thyroid signaling interact to influence energy, mood, cognition, and immune function. AI evaluates these interactions over time rather than in isolation, revealing patterns that traditional testing often misses. Early stabilization of hormonal rhythms prevents cascading dysfunction that would otherwise appear unrelated.

What makes AI uniquely effective is its systems-level perspective. Rather than addressing symptoms individually, it protects the architecture that keeps the body adaptable. When regulatory systems are stable, the body tolerates stress, heals efficiently, and resists disease. When regulation erodes, even minor stressors produce exaggerated damage. AI identifies erosion early and directs attention to the systems that matter most, preserving health without aggressive intervention. Importantly, protecting regulatory systems does not require extreme optimization. Overcontrol can be as harmful as neglect. AI emphasizes ranges rather than targets, resilience rather than rigidity. It recognizes that variability is normal and healthy, as long as recovery remains efficient. This approach aligns with long-term sustainability, especially for aging adults who need consistency rather than intensity.

By shifting prevention toward regulation rather than reaction, AI changes the entire trajectory of aging. Chronic disease becomes less about inevitable decline and more about maintaining internal balance. This chapter establishes why protecting regulatory systems is the most efficient way to reduce disease burden and why AI is uniquely suited to perform this role quietly in the background of everyday life.

Stability Before Symptoms

When Daniel turned sixty-four, he felt unsettled despite a clean bill of health. His doctor reassured him that his labs were normal, but Daniel noticed subtle changes he couldn't explain. Stress lingered longer than it used to. Sleep felt lighter. Minor illnesses took more time to resolve. None of these issues rose to the level of complaint, yet together they created a sense that his body was working harder to stay balanced.

At the suggestion of a colleague, Daniel began using an AI-based health monitoring platform focused on long-term trends. The early summaries did not alarm him. Instead, they revealed something more subtle. His autonomic nervous system showed reduced variability during periods of prolonged stress. Sleep fragmentation correlated with inflammatory instability. Metabolic recovery after exertion slowed incrementally each year. His body was still functioning well, but its regulatory systems were losing flexibility.

Rather than recommending drastic change, the AI platform highlighted stability as the priority. Daniel adjusted his schedule to protect consistent sleep timing, reduced late-day stress exposure, and moderated workout intensity without reducing activity. He also learned to recognize early signs of overload rather than pushing through them.

Over the next year, the data shifted. Recovery curves shortened. Sleep architecture improved. Inflammatory fluctuations stabilized. Daniel felt calmer and more resilient, though he had not consciously "fixed" anything. His clinician reviewed the summaries and agreed that no medical intervention was needed. Regulation had been restored naturally.

Several years later, Daniel watched peers navigate new diagnoses that seemed to arrive suddenly. He recognized the familiar signs they described from his own past. The difference was not luck. It was attention. By protecting regulation before symptoms demanded action, Daniel preserved health quietly and efficiently. Aging continued, but disease did not follow. Stability, he realized, had been the most powerful intervention of all.

Chapter 6

How AI Reduces Long-Term Disease Burden by Preventing System Overload

Chronic disease is rarely caused by a single failure. It emerges when the body is pushed beyond its capacity to recover, adapt, and rebalance. This state is best described as system overload. Overload occurs when stress accumulates faster than the body can resolve it, forcing biological systems to operate continuously in emergency mode. Artificial intelligence plays a critical role in preventing chronic disease by identifying overload early and guiding interventions that reduce cumulative strain before permanent damage occurs.

System overload develops gradually and often invisibly. Stress hormones remain elevated longer than intended. Inflammatory responses fail to fully resolve. Sleep becomes lighter and less restorative. Metabolic processes lose efficiency. Individually, these changes may appear insignificant. Together, they create a state where the body is constantly compensating without relief. AI identifies overload by detecting prolonged deviations from baseline rather than acute spikes. This distinction is essential because chronic disease is driven more by duration than intensity. One of the most important ways AI detects overload is by analyzing recovery capacity. Recovery is not the absence of stress, but the ability to return to equilibrium after stress occurs. AI tracks how long it takes for physiological markers such as heart rate variability, resting heart rate, glucose stability, inflammation indicators, and sleep architecture to normalize after disruption. When recovery slows consistently, it signals that the system is nearing overload. Acting at this stage prevents progression to dysfunction.

AI also identifies cumulative stress across domains that are often treated separately. Psychological stress, physical exertion, poor sleep, metabolic strain, and environmental factors interact synergistically. A body may tolerate any one of these stressors individually, but not all simultaneously. AI integrates data across these domains to reveal total load rather than isolated inputs. This integrated perspective explains why individuals sometimes develop chronic disease despite appearing healthy by conventional measures. Their total load exceeds their adaptive capacity.

Preventing overload requires restraint as much as action. Many well-intentioned health efforts inadvertently increase stress by adding complexity, rigidity, or excessive intensity. AI counters this by identifying when additional intervention would worsen overload rather than relieve it. Sometimes the most effective prevention strategy is subtraction: reducing training volume, simplifying routines, stabilizing schedules, or prioritizing rest. AI supports these decisions with data, reducing guilt and uncertainty.

Another advantage of AI-driven overload prevention is personalization. Adaptive capacity varies widely between individuals and changes with age. What one person tolerates easily may overwhelm another. AI learns each individual's limits by observing responses over time rather than assuming universal thresholds. This prevents comparisons and encourages self-referenced decision-making, which is essential for sustainable aging.

AI also helps prevent overload by identifying compounding patterns. For example, poor sleep may amplify metabolic instability, which increases inflammation, which strains cardiovascular regulation. AI detects these feedback loops early and identifies where breaking the loop produces the greatest relief. Addressing a single leverage point often reduces strain across multiple systems, making prevention efficient rather than burdensome.

Importantly, preventing overload does not mean avoiding challenge. The body requires stress to maintain strength, resilience, and adaptability. AI distinguishes productive stress from destructive accumulation by evaluating recovery quality.

Stress followed by recovery builds capacity. Stress without recovery depletes it. This distinction allows individuals to remain active, engaged, and challenged without crossing into chronic strain.

Over time, preventing system overload preserves optionality. When regulatory systems remain intact, the body retains the ability to respond to illness, injury, or life changes. Chronic disease reduces this flexibility, forcing rigid management strategies. AI-driven prevention keeps options open by maintaining capacity rather than reacting to failure.

Ultimately, AI reduces long-term disease burden by acting as a load manager for the body. It does not eliminate stress, aging, or change. It ensures that these forces remain within the body's ability to adapt. This chapter establishes why overload is the hidden driver behind most chronic disease and how AI prevents decline by protecting recovery before exhaustion becomes pathology.

Learning When to Stop Pushing

When Victor turned sixty, he believed effort was the solution to everything. If he felt tired, he trained harder. If stress increased, he worked longer. If sleep suffered, he ignored it and pushed through. This mindset had served him well for decades, but subtle changes were emerging. He caught colds more easily. Injuries lingered. Fatigue no longer resolved with a weekend of rest. Still, Victor refused to slow down, convinced that discipline was the answer.

At his wife's insistence, Victor joined a preventive health program that used AI to analyze long-term physiological trends. He expected criticism for not doing enough. Instead, the data revealed something unexpected. His body was overloaded. Recovery metrics showed prolonged suppression after stress. Sleep fragmentation persisted even during low-activity periods. Inflammation markers failed to return to baseline. The problem was not lack of effort, but lack of relief.

The AI system recommended fewer changes than Victor anticipated. It suggested shorter training sessions with built-in recovery days, consistent sleep timing, and reduced late-evening stimulation. Victor resisted at first, viewing these adjustments as weakness. But the data was clear. On weeks when he followed the guidance, recovery improved. Energy stabilized. Minor aches faded more quickly.

Over the next year, Victor learned a new relationship with effort. He remained active, but no longer relentless. He listened to early signs of overload rather than dismissing them. The AI summaries showed growing resilience rather than decline. When Victor's longtime training partner developed joint degeneration and chronic fatigue, Victor recognized the familiar pattern. He had been on the same path.

By sixty-five, Victor felt stronger than he had at sixty, not because he pushed harder, but because he stopped pushing past recovery. Chronic disease had not been avoided through intensity, but through balance. AI had not told him to do more. It had taught him when enough was enough. That lesson, he realized, had preserved not just his health, but his future.

Chapter 7

How AI Creates a Continuous Prevention Loop That Adapts as You Age

Chronic disease prevention fails most often not because people lack information, but because health strategies do not evolve as the body changes. Aging is dynamic, yet most prevention efforts are static. Advice given at forty is repeated at fifty and ignored at sixty, even though biology shifts continuously across these decades. Artificial intelligence solves this mismatch by creating a continuous prevention loop that updates in real time, learning from the body's responses and adjusting guidance as conditions change. This adaptive loop is what transforms prevention from a phase of life into a lifelong system.

At the core of this loop is feedback. The body is constantly communicating through physiological signals, but without interpretation those signals go unheard. AI listens continuously, comparing present patterns to past baselines and expected trajectories. When the body adapts well, the system recognizes stability and avoids unnecessary intervention. When adaptation weakens, AI detects early drift and adjusts recommendations before damage accumulates. This loop prevents both neglect and overreaction, maintaining balance across years rather than responding to crises.

A key advantage of continuous prevention is that it respects the nonlinear nature of aging. Health does not decline in straight lines. It fluctuates with seasons, stress, illness, and life events. AI accommodates this variability by evaluating trends rather than moments. Temporary disruption does not trigger alarm, while persistent deviation prompts attention. This distinction prevents burnout and fear-driven behavior while ensuring that real risk is not ignored.

As individuals move from their forties into their fifties and beyond, the prevention loop naturally shifts focus. Early on, the emphasis may be metabolic efficiency and stress resilience. Later, it may prioritize mobility, cardiovascular stability, cognitive preservation, or recovery capacity. AI recognizes these transitions automatically, guided by data rather than assumptions. This removes the burden of decision-making from the individual, allowing prevention to remain relevant without constant re-education.

Another strength of the prevention loop is that it reinforces behaviors that work and deemphasizes those that do not. Many people persist with routines long after they stop producing benefit. AI evaluates outcomes rather than intentions. If a habit improves recovery, stability, or resilience, it remains part of the loop. If it increases strain or produces diminishing returns, the system adapts. This prevents stagnation and keeps prevention aligned with reality rather than ideology.

The loop also protects against cumulative blind spots. Over time, people normalize subtle decline and adjust expectations downward. AI does not normalize decline; it tracks it. By preserving historical context, the system highlights changes that would otherwise fade into the background. This is especially important later in life, when small losses compound more quickly. Continuous prevention ensures that no decade quietly erodes the foundation laid in the previous one.

Importantly, this loop operates quietly. Effective prevention does not dominate attention or identity. AI reduces the need for constant monitoring by identifying when attention is required and when it is not. This allows individuals to live fully while prevention functions in the background, intervening only when necessary. Health becomes a managed process rather than a daily concern.

The continuous prevention loop also strengthens trust. Because recommendations are reinforced by observable outcomes, confidence grows over time. Individuals learn how their bodies respond, which signals matter most, and when intervention is worthwhile. This relationship reduces dependence on external reassurance and replaces it with informed self-awareness supported by data.

Ultimately, AI-driven prevention succeeds because it mirrors how the body itself operates: continuously, adaptively, and contextually. Rather than imposing rigid rules, it responds to change. Rather than reacting to failure, it anticipates drift. This chapter completes the prevention framework by showing how AI sustains health across decades, ensuring that chronic disease prevention remains effective not just today, but for the rest of life.

A System That Aged With Him

When Robert turned fifty-two, he decided to take prevention seriously. He had watched his father's health decline rapidly in his sixties and wanted a different future. At first, Robert approached health with enthusiasm, tracking metrics obsessively and experimenting with routines. For a while, improvements came quickly. But as years passed, life intervened. Career pressures increased, family responsibilities shifted, and the rigid system he had built became harder to maintain.

At fifty-six, Robert transitioned to an AI-based prevention platform that emphasized adaptation rather than control. The system did not overwhelm him with daily demands. Instead, it quietly monitored trends and provided periodic summaries. When stress increased, it adjusted expectations. When recovery slowed, it suggested rest rather than effort. The system evolved as Robert did, without requiring constant engagement.

In his early sixties, Robert noticed that the focus of the guidance shifted. Where once it emphasized metabolic efficiency and workload balance, it now highlighted sleep stability, joint recovery, and cardiovascular resilience. The changes felt natural rather than forced. He trusted the system because it had proven responsive over time.

At sixty-seven, Robert faced a health scare when a close friend suffered a sudden cardiac event. Reviewing his own data, Robert saw years of preserved stability. His prevention loop had identified and corrected small deviations long before they escalated. His clinician confirmed that his risk profile remained low for his age, not because he had avoided aging, but because he had adapted with it.

Looking back, Robert realized the most valuable aspect of the system was not prediction or control, but continuity.

Prevention had not been a phase he outgrew or abandoned. It had grown with him. AI had not frozen him in time; it had allowed him to move forward without leaving his health behind. The future no longer felt uncertain. It felt managed, quietly and intelligently, one adaptive loop at a time.

Chapter 8

How AI Shifts Health From Crisis Management to Lifelong Stability

For most people, healthcare begins only when something goes wrong. Symptoms appear, tests are ordered, and treatment follows. This reactive model has defined modern medicine for generations, yet it is poorly suited for aging populations and chronic disease prevention. Artificial intelligence enables a fundamental shift away from crisis management and toward lifelong stability by identifying risk before disruption occurs and guiding the body back to balance without waiting for failure. This chapter explains how AI transforms health from a series of emergencies into a continuously stabilized system.

Crisis-based healthcare is effective for acute events but inefficient for long-term health. It intervenes after damage has accumulated and often addresses symptoms rather than causes. By contrast, AI-driven prevention operates upstream. It monitors the conditions that make crises likely and adjusts them early. This does not eliminate illness or injury entirely, but it dramatically reduces frequency, severity, and recovery time. Health becomes something that is maintained rather than rescued. One of the most important ways AI enables this shift is by identifying fragility before it becomes visible.

Fragility develops when systems lose redundancy and adaptability. Minor disruptions that were once inconsequential begin to produce outsized effects. AI detects this loss by tracking recovery efficiency, variability tolerance, and stability margins. When fragility increases, AI responds by strengthening foundations rather than waiting for collapse. This approach preserves independence and reduces the emotional and financial cost of late-stage care.

AI also reframes the concept of risk. Traditional medicine categorizes people as healthy or sick, with little recognition of the spectrum between. AI recognizes gradations. It understands that most people spend decades in a preclinical state where outcomes are highly modifiable. By operating in this space, AI reduces the likelihood that individuals will ever cross into irreversible disease. Stability becomes the goal rather than perfection, and risk becomes something to be managed rather than feared.

Another advantage of AI-driven stability is its cumulative effect. Small improvements sustained over years produce exponential benefit. Reduced inflammation preserves vascular health. Stable metabolism protects cognition. Consistent recovery maintains mobility. AI tracks these compounding gains, reinforcing behaviors that quietly extend healthspan. This long-view perspective is difficult for humans to maintain but natural for AI systems designed to evaluate trends over decades.

Stability-oriented health also improves decision-making during inevitable disruptions. Illness, injury, surgery, and stress are unavoidable aspects of life. When the body is stable, these events are absorbed and resolved more effectively. AI prepares individuals for these moments by preserving reserve capacity. Rather than scrambling after disruption, recovery becomes smoother and faster. This resilience is the true measure of health in later life.

Importantly, shifting away from crisis does not mean ignoring warning signs. It means responding proportionately. AI distinguishes between transient noise and meaningful signal, preventing both neglect and overreaction. This measured response reduces anxiety and unnecessary intervention while ensuring that genuine risk is addressed promptly. Over time, trust develops, allowing individuals to disengage emotionally while remaining protected biologically.

The financial and emotional implications of this shift are profound. Chronic disease crises often lead to cascading costs, loss of independence, and caregiver burden. By reducing disease burden before crises emerge, AI supports not only individual health but family stability and quality of life. Aging becomes less disruptive and more predictable, allowing planning rather than reaction.

Ultimately, AI-driven stability represents a new health paradigm. It aligns medicine with biology, prevention with reality, and aging with continuity rather than collapse. This chapter positions AI not as a diagnostic tool, but as a stabilizing force that keeps the body within its adaptive range across decades. Health is no longer something to rescue when it fails. It becomes something to quietly protect every day.

The Emergency That Never Came

When Linda turned sixty-five, she expected health to become a series of surprises. She had watched friends cycle through emergencies that seemed to appear suddenly and derail lives overnight. Falls, heart scares, autoimmune flares, and unexplained fatigue became common conversation topics. Linda assumed that this was simply what aging looked like.

Several years earlier, Linda had begun using an AI-driven health monitoring system focused on long-term stability rather than diagnosis. At first, it felt unremarkable. The system did not issue warnings or demand action. It simply tracked patterns and suggested modest adjustments when needed. Linda trusted it because it never overreacted. In her late sixties, Linda experienced a period of intense stress when her spouse underwent surgery. Sleep suffered, routines broke down, and anxiety lingered. In the past, this kind of disruption might have triggered cascading health issues. Instead, the AI system adjusted expectations, emphasized recovery, and highlighted early signs of strain before they escalated. Linda responded with rest rather than panic.

Months later, her clinician reviewed the data and noted something remarkable. Despite significant stress, Linda's physiological stability had been preserved. Recovery metrics remained strong. Inflammatory volatility stayed controlled. Cardiovascular resilience held steady. Linda had not avoided stress, but she had avoided crisis.

At seventy-two, Linda realized something else had changed. She no longer lived with quiet dread of the next health emergency. Years had passed without dramatic events, not because she was lucky, but because her health had been stabilized long before problems could erupt. AI had not predicted disasters. It had prevented conditions that allow disasters to form.

Looking ahead, Linda felt calm rather than anxious. Aging continued, but it no longer felt like a countdown. Health had shifted from something fragile to something supported. The emergencies she once expected never came, not because life was perfect, but because stability had quietly done its work.

Chapter 9

How AI Preserves Independence by Extending Functional Healthspan

Longevity without independence is not the goal of prevention. Living longer only matters if the added years remain functional, mobile, cognitively intact, and self-directed. Chronic disease erodes independence gradually, not only through life-threatening events but through incremental losses in strength, clarity, endurance, and confidence. Artificial intelligence contributes to long-term independence by extending healthspan, the period of life lived with full functional capacity. This chapter explores how AI protects mobility, cognition, metabolic stability, and resilience to preserve autonomy well into later decades.

Functional decline rarely begins with dramatic illness. It begins with subtle reductions in strength, balance, recovery speed, and mental clarity. These small losses compound over time, leading to reduced activity, social withdrawal, and increased vulnerability to injury or disease. AI identifies these early changes by tracking performance metrics across multiple systems. Reaction time, gait variability, heart rate recovery, sleep quality, glucose stability, and inflammatory trends all contribute to a comprehensive view of functional health. When patterns begin to drift, AI highlights them before they manifest as visible decline.

One of the most important aspects of functional healthspan is mobility. Loss of strength and balance increases fall risk, which is one of the most significant predictors of long-term disability. AI monitors musculoskeletal strain, recovery from exertion, and coordination patterns to detect early instability. By identifying when recovery slows or asymmetries develop, AI allows corrective adjustments before injury occurs. Preventing the first fall is far more effective than recovering from one.

Cognitive independence is equally critical. Subtle changes in attention, memory consistency, and processing speed often precede diagnosable impairment by years. AI correlates cognitive performance data with sleep patterns, cardiovascular stability, metabolic efficiency, and stress load. This systems-level perspective identifies whether cognitive fluctuation is transient or part of a larger trend. Early adjustments in sleep, recovery, and metabolic balance can preserve clarity and delay or prevent decline.

Metabolic stability underpins both physical and cognitive independence. Blood sugar variability, inflammatory fluctuations, and cardiovascular strain all influence energy and endurance. AI continuously evaluates these interactions, reinforcing behaviors that sustain stable energy rather than short-term spikes. Over time, this stability preserves capacity for daily activities and reduces fatigue-driven inactivity, which is a major contributor to late-life decline.

Resilience also determines independence. Illness, surgery, or emotional stress are unavoidable. The ability to recover quickly from these events defines long-term autonomy. AI strengthens resilience by maintaining reserve capacity across systems. When recovery metrics begin to shrink, AI encourages proportionate adjustments that rebuild capacity before crisis forces intervention.

Psychologically, preserving independence requires confidence. Fear of decline often accelerates withdrawal and inactivity. AI reduces uncertainty by providing clarity. Individuals who understand their trajectory are more likely to stay engaged, active, and proactive. Confidence supports participation, which in turn reinforces strength and cognition.

Importantly, extending healthspan is not about extreme optimization. It is about consistency. AI encourages sustainable habits that compound over years rather than temporary programs that fade. By reinforcing what works and identifying when adaptation is needed, AI maintains momentum without exhaustion. Ultimately, AI protects independence by preventing the silent erosion that leads to dependency. Healthspan extension is achieved not through dramatic breakthroughs but through continuous stabilization. This chapter highlights how AI shifts the focus of longevity from survival to capability, ensuring that added years remain meaningful and self-directed.

The Years That Stayed His

Miguel had always valued self-sufficiency. At sixty-eight, he still drove himself to appointments, maintained his garden, and enjoyed long walks with his grandchildren. Yet he noticed subtle shifts. Rising from chairs felt slightly harder. His balance wavered on uneven ground. Names occasionally slipped from memory. None of these changes were dramatic, but they unsettled him.

Several years earlier, Miguel's daughter had encouraged him to adopt an AI-based health monitoring system focused on functional trends. Miguel agreed reluctantly, skeptical of technology. The system tracked recovery patterns, gait stability, sleep quality, and metabolic consistency. For a long time, the reports were reassuring. Gradually, however, they highlighted early signs of declining balance recovery and prolonged post-exertion fatigue. Rather than alarming him, the system suggested modest adjustments. Miguel incorporated targeted balance exercises, moderated exertion intensity, and protected consistent sleep timing. Within months, recovery metrics improved. Gait variability stabilized. Confidence returned. Miguel felt stronger not because he was younger, but because he had intervened early.

When a close friend suffered a hip fracture after a fall, Miguel recognized how quickly independence could be lost. Reviewing his own data, he saw years of preserved stability. The early adjustments he had once questioned had prevented larger consequences.

At seventy-four, Miguel remained active and autonomous. He still drove, gardened, and traveled independently. Aging continued, but dependency did not follow. AI had not made him invincible. It had preserved the subtle capacities that make independence possible. The years ahead felt like extensions of life rather than contractions of ability. The years, as he often said, had stayed his.

Chapter 10

The Smart Aging Blueprint: A Lifelong AI-Guided System for Disease-Free Living

Chronic disease prevention is not a single intervention, a short-term program, or a seasonal commitment. It is a structure that must adapt as the body evolves across decades. The Smart Aging Blueprint represents the integration of everything explored in this book: early detection, regulatory protection, overload prevention, continuous feedback, resilience preservation, and independence maintenance. Artificial intelligence makes this blueprint sustainable by transforming prevention from effort into architecture. This chapter unifies the concepts into a lifelong, adaptive system designed to protect health from midlife through advanced age.

The foundation of the Smart Aging Blueprint is awareness without obsession. Health data must inform, not dominate. AI accomplishes this by filtering noise from signal, highlighting meaningful shifts while ignoring temporary fluctuations. Instead of daily micromanagement, individuals receive periodic clarity. This preserves emotional energy and prevents health from becoming a source of stress. When intervention is needed, it is proportionate and specific. When stability is present, life proceeds uninterrupted.

The blueprint begins with baseline mapping. Every body has a unique starting point shaped by genetics, history, stress exposure, and lifestyle patterns. AI establishes personal baselines across metabolic, cardiovascular, inflammatory, neurological, sleep, and recovery domains. These baselines replace generic norms with individualized context. As years pass, comparisons are made against personal trajectory rather than population averages. This personalized benchmarking allows early course correction without waiting for universal thresholds to be crossed.

The second pillar of the blueprint is regulatory reinforcement. As described in earlier chapters, chronic disease emerges when regulation deteriorates. The blueprint prioritizes strengthening the systems that maintain balance: autonomic stability, metabolic flexibility, sleep architecture, inflammatory resolution, and hormonal rhythm. AI monitors these systems continuously and recommends minimal adjustments that preserve resilience. Over time, reinforced regulation becomes protective armor against disease.

The third pillar is load management. Aging bodies tolerate stress differently across decades. AI evaluates cumulative load from physical exertion, psychological strain, environmental factors, and recovery patterns. When overload approaches, adjustments are introduced before breakdown occurs. This prevents the silent accumulation of damage that leads to chronic illness. The blueprint does not eliminate stress; it ensures stress remains productive rather than destructive.

The fourth pillar is compounding stability. Small improvements, sustained consistently, create exponential benefit. AI identifies which behaviors stabilize multiple systems simultaneously and reinforces them. These may include sleep consistency, balanced activity cycles, metabolic rhythm alignment, and stress recovery practices. Because the system is adaptive, behaviors evolve as needs change. What stabilizes a forty-five-year-old may differ from what stabilizes a seventy-year-old. AI recognizes these transitions and adjusts focus seamlessly.

The fifth pillar is resilience preservation. Health is not defined by the absence of stress but by the ability to recover from it. AI tracks reserve capacity across domains, ensuring that unexpected events do not overwhelm systems. By maintaining resilience margins, the blueprint reduces the severity of illness, speeds recovery, and preserves independence. The sixth pillar is longitudinal continuity. Many prevention efforts fail because they are episodic. The Smart Aging Blueprint is continuous. It does not restart every January or after every medical visit. It evolves quietly over years. AI ensures that progress is not lost when life becomes busy or chaotic. The system remembers history even when individuals cannot.

Importantly, the Smart Aging Blueprint is not about perfection. It is about direction. Trends matter more than isolated events. Stability matters more than intensity. Consistency matters more than enthusiasm. AI reinforces these principles by evaluating patterns rather than moments. This reduces burnout and increases sustainability.

As individuals move into later decades, the blueprint naturally shifts toward independence preservation. Mobility, cognitive clarity, energy stability, and cardiovascular resilience become priorities. AI anticipates these shifts by recognizing early declines and reinforcing protective behaviors before functional loss becomes visible.

Ultimately, the Smart Aging Blueprint represents a partnership between biology and intelligence. It allows aging to unfold without unnecessary acceleration. Chronic disease becomes less likely not because it is feared, but because its precursors are managed quietly and intelligently. The blueprint is not a promise of immortality. It is a commitment to trajectory. With AI guiding course correction, aging becomes something to navigate rather than endure.

Designing the Last Decades Well

Evelyn was fifty-three when she decided she did not want to leave her health to chance. She had watched her parents' later years become defined by medications, limitations, and dependency. Nothing catastrophic had happened suddenly. Decline had crept in quietly, year by year, until options narrowed. Evelyn wanted a different path.

She began by establishing a baseline through an AI-driven health platform that analyzed her historical records, wearable data, sleep patterns, metabolic responses, and cardiovascular markers. The first report did not show disease. It showed trajectory. Recovery after stress was lengthening. Sleep consistency was eroding. Glucose variability spiked during work pressure. The trends were subtle, but clear.

Instead of reacting dramatically, Evelyn committed to structure. She aligned sleep timing more consistently, adjusted her work schedule to reduce late-night strain, incorporated moderate strength training rather than high-intensity sessions, and built recovery days into her routine. AI tracked her responses over months. Recovery curves improved. Inflammatory volatility decreased. Energy stabilized. At sixty, Evelyn encountered a major stressor when her spouse was hospitalized unexpectedly. Years earlier, such an event might have destabilized her health. This time, her resilience held. AI flagged temporary strain but showed preserved recovery capacity. She adjusted slightly, rested intentionally, and returned to baseline without lingering dysfunction.

At sixty-eight, Evelyn reviewed nearly fifteen years of data. The trajectory that once pointed toward accelerated decline had flattened into stability. Her clinician remarked that her physiological markers resembled those of someone years younger. More importantly, she felt capable. She traveled independently, maintained strength, and engaged mentally without fear of fragility.

By seventy-five, Evelyn realized that the most powerful part of her blueprint had not been any single adjustment. It had been continuity. There had been no dramatic turning points, no emergency interventions, no sudden reversals. There had only been steady course correction guided by intelligence and reinforced by discipline.

When friends spoke of surprise diagnoses and rapid decline, Evelyn felt gratitude not for luck, but for foresight. She had designed her later decades intentionally. The last chapters of her life were unfolding not as damage control, but as extension. The blueprint had worked quietly in the background, ensuring that aging did not steal what she valued most: clarity, mobility, independence, and peace.

Epilogue

The Future You Are Already Building

Aging does not begin in the future. It is happening now, quietly, whether you are forty-five or seventy-five. Every choice, every recovery cycle, every period of stress or stability contributes to a trajectory that unfolds across decades. What this book has demonstrated is not that disease can be magically eliminated, but that its path can be reshaped. Artificial intelligence offers something previous generations never had: visibility into the patterns that determine how aging unfolds long before decline becomes visible. The future version of you is not a mystery. It is a continuation of your present trajectory, and that trajectory can be guided.

The most important insight from this journey is that chronic disease is rarely sudden. It is cumulative. It grows from unresolved stress, unstable regulation, silent inflammation, metabolic drift, and eroding resilience. These forces do not appear dramatically; they accumulate quietly. The tragedy of traditional healthcare is not incompetence but timing. It intervenes after thresholds are crossed rather than when direction begins to shift. AI changes timing. It extends the window in which intervention is simple, sustainable, and effective. You now understand that prevention is not intensity.

It is continuity. It is the preservation of regulatory systems, the management of cumulative load, the reinforcement of resilience, and the extension of healthspan through steady stabilization. These concepts are not dramatic, and that is precisely why they work. Sustainable aging is quiet. It rarely announces itself. It simply avoids unnecessary decline.

One of the most powerful psychological shifts AI enables is moving from fear to foresight. Fear reacts to symptoms. Foresight observes trajectory. Fear waits for crisis. Foresight adjusts course early. When individuals see their own trends and understand how small adjustments alter outcomes, anxiety decreases. Health becomes something navigable rather than unpredictable. Confidence replaces dread because direction is visible.

It is important to understand that the Smart Aging Blueprint is not a technological dependency. It is a framework. AI serves as an interpreter of signals, but the responsibility remains human. Data does not act. You act. Technology does not replace wisdom; it enhances it. The goal is not to surrender judgment to algorithms, but to refine judgment with clarity that was previously inaccessible.

Over time, prevention becomes identity-neutral. It is no longer a project or a program. It becomes background architecture supporting daily life. The most successful individuals in this model rarely think of themselves as optimizing. They simply respond to signals proportionately. When recovery slows, they rest. When load accumulates, they subtract. When stability improves, they continue. This rhythm mirrors how biology prefers to operate.

Aging will always involve change. Strength shifts. Hormones fluctuate. Recovery capacity narrows. But decline is not the same as deterioration. With continuous feedback and adaptive correction, change can remain gradual rather than catastrophic. Chronic disease becomes less likely not because you eliminate risk entirely, but because you refuse to allow small deviations to compound unchecked.

The final lesson of this book is that time is leverage. Every year of stabilized regulation compounds. Every avoided cascade prevents additional cascades. The earlier the blueprint begins, the greater the dividend. But it is never too late to alter trajectory. Even in later decades, stabilizing recovery and reinforcing regulation produces meaningful improvement.

You are not waiting for the future. You are constructing it. Every period of stable sleep, balanced load, metabolic consistency, and resilient recovery becomes a building block. AI simply illuminates the structure as it forms. The rest is patience and continuity.

The future you is already emerging from today's patterns. The question is not whether aging will occur, but whether it will be accelerated by neglect or stabilized by foresight. You now possess the framework to choose the latter.

The Man Who Met Himself at Eighty

When James was fifty-eight, he avoided thinking about eighty. It felt distant, abstract, and irrelevant to daily life. He focused on work, family, and short-term goals. Health was something he addressed only when symptoms forced attention. But subtle changes were accumulating. Recovery slowed. Energy dipped. Sleep fractured more easily. None of it seemed urgent.

After reading about AI-driven prevention, James decided to experiment. He began tracking patterns and reviewing trend summaries monthly. The first year revealed something surprising. His stress recovery curves were lengthening gradually. Inflammatory fluctuations correlated with poor sleep. His metabolic variability increased during travel and deadlines. These were not crises. They were signals.

James committed not to dramatic overhaul, but to consistency. He stabilized sleep timing, moderated workload intensity, and built recovery days into his schedule. The adjustments felt modest, almost insignificant. Yet within a year, his data stabilized. He felt subtly better but did not consider it transformational.

At sixty-five, James experienced a difficult year. A business setback and family stress disrupted routines. Instead of spiraling into fatigue and dysfunction, he reviewed his long-term data. He saw preserved resilience from years of stabilization. He adjusted temporarily, restored sleep consistency, reduced unnecessary load, and returned to baseline. What might once have become chronic dysfunction resolved within months.

At seventy-two, James reviewed nearly fifteen years of health data. The trajectory was not perfect, but it was stable. Small dips appeared and recovered. There were no cascading declines. His clinician noted preserved cardiovascular health and cognitive clarity unusual for his age. James realized that the compounding effect of small, sustained corrections had reshaped his later decades.

When James turned eighty, he reflected on the man he had been at fifty-eight. He imagined what might have happened had he ignored those early signals. He likely would have continued pushing through fatigue, dismissing sleep disruption, and normalizing subtle decline. The difference between that imagined eighty-year-old and the man he had become was not genetics or luck. It was trajectory.

At eighty, James still walked independently, traveled occasionally, and engaged mentally without fear. He did not feel frozen in youth. He felt preserved in capacity. Aging had continued, but collapse had not followed.

One evening, sitting quietly after dinner, James thought about time differently. He had once believed that eighty was something that happened to you. Now he understood that eighty was something you prepared for. The man he met at eighty was not a surprise. He was the predictable outcome of years of quiet course correction.

James smiled at the realization that he had, in a sense, met himself decades earlier. The future had never been sudden. It had been constructed daily, stabilized yearly, and protected patiently. Artificial intelligence had not changed his destiny. It had clarified his direction. The rest had been consistency.

www.ingramcontent.com/pod-product-compliance
Lightning Source LLC
LaVergne TN
LVHW022022200926
848481LV00007B/2500
* 9 7 9 8 2 9 5 6 6 4 9 6 0 *